British Association of Holist

A Guide to Plants
Poisonous to Horses

Keith Allison

VETERINARY ADVISER
Christopher Day MRCVS

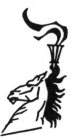

J.A. Allen
London

British Library Cataloguing in Publication Data
A catalogue record for this book is available from the British Library.

ISBN 0.85131.698.0

Published in Great Britain in 1997 by
J. A. Allen & Company Limited
1 Lower Grosvenor Place
London SW1W 0EL

Typeset by Textype Typesetters, Cambridge
Printed by Dah Hua Printing Co. Ltd., Hong Kong

Edited by Elizabeth O'Beirne-Ranelagh
Designed by Nancy Lawrence

Acknowledgements

The author wishes to acknowledge the following, used as
reference material in order to ensure a high level of accuracy
of entries. They are also recommended for further reading.

Herbs and healing plants by Dieter Podlech (Collins)
The concise British flora by W Keble Martin (BCA)
Poisonous plants in Britain by M Cooper and A Johnson (HMSO)
New herbal by Richard Mabey (Penguin)
Herbal medicine by Rudolf Fritz Weiss (Beaconsfield)

Contents

Introduction

Traditional agricultural practice allowed and encouraged a much greater variety of pasture species to exist than is the case today. Before the 1940s, a meadow may have contained well over a hundred different varieties of herbage, compared with perhaps ten species in a modern pasture.

As the number of different species of plants in the countryside declined (largely through the use of nitrogenous fertilisers), so did general knowledge about their effect on animals. Many potentially toxic plants disappeared along with beneficial species, and so it became less important to be able to identify them as they became less of a threat to livestock.

The trend away from extensive use of chemicals together with the employment of more traditional methods of farming means that species diversity may increase. Along with the nutritional benefits that this brings, there is also a risk, in that many potentially poisonous species of wild plants may return, together with those which, although not outright poisons in themselves, may be toxic to some degree. It is becoming more important, therefore, to be able to identify a wider range of potentially dangerous herbage in order to assess the risk for the grazing horse.

Most horse-owners know the dangers of, and can identify, plants such as ragwort, yew, laburnum and bracken, which are the most common cause of poisoning in horses. There are, however, many hundreds of others which although not generally thought of as dangerous can in theory be toxic to animals. The risk of poisoning from some species is difficult to assess scientifically, simply because experimental work has not been carried out to ascertain the precise poisonous principles. In these circumstances it is necessary to resort to properly documented cases of poisoning involving the species concerned.

Listed below are 55 plants which are commonly regarded as being poisonous in their own right. A profile of each is given together with its prevalence, poisonous principle and symptoms. Information on treatment is not given as it would be beyond the intended scope of this booklet. If a horse is suspected of having ingested toxic herbage, veterinary assistance should be obtained without delay. If the herbage can be positively identified by giving a description of the plant, together with the symptoms, over the telephone, advice may be given on first aid measures which should be followed before the veterinary surgeon arrives. Information and specialist advice in cases of poisoning is available for veterinary surgeons from the Veterinary Poisons Information Unit in Leeds (see p. 69).

Poisoning is generally thought of as being a dramatic event, as indeed it can be, but it may also be a question of degree. It is thought that many horses, along with other grazing animals, often suffer from the effects of mild toxicity, which may go unnoticed. Non-specific allergies, weight loss, lethargy, mild digestive problems and others may not be associated by the owner or veterinary surgeon with toxins, especially if the symptoms are relatively mild.

If a horse is suspected of having been poisoned, not only should the grazing be taken into account, but also other sources of toxins. The possibility of cumulative over-dose of synthetic feed supplements or contaminants in herbal or other 'natural' products should not be overlooked. It should be mentioned here that, in general, supplements are over-used, and that they should only be given in specific circumstances and after careful consideration.*

Maintaining a healthy balance of species in pasture is central to reducing the risk of problems arising from the horse eating plants which are either outright poisons or toxic in certain circumstances.* In general horses will not poison themselves unless the floristic balance is seriously distorted. The highest risk is in weed-infested, horse-sick paddocks where horses are driven to feed on plants which normally they would either avoid completely, or take in substantially lower amounts. Drought conditions can increase the risk of poisoning because some species may have a higher concentration of toxins at this time. Some species are more toxic in wet weather. Some undesirable plants such as buttercups and docks, and including high-risk species such as ragwort, are colonisers which increase their number with over-grazing – as desirable

* The BAHNM will advise – see p. 69.

species decline, so more of the undesirable species may be eaten. Also animals grazing on poor pasture are more likely to succumb to the plant poisons. Whilst many plants in Britain are known to be poisonous, reported cases of fatalities through ingestion of toxic herbage are fortunately rare. It is very difficult to obtain precise figures, however, because many animals that are poisoned may not be reported because the condition is misdiagnosed and/or the animal recovers.

Most toxic plants are too pungent or too bitter for a horse to ingest them, unless he is craving something or is exceptionally hungry. There are many plants, therefore, which are potentially toxic for which no cases of poisoning have been reported.

Plant chemistry

The principle in medicine that certain substances may either be poisonous or curative, depending on the amount taken, is well known. As we have seen, traditional pastures were rich in herbal species, many of which in isolation may be toxic to some degree, but may also be beneficial to health when taken in proper amounts as part of an holistic nutritional profile.

What makes a particular plant attractive to a domesticated horse depends on a number of factors relevant to the particular situation. It is plain, however, that in the natural order of things feral horses instinctively know what is good for them and will select a diet accordingly. It is clear also that all ingredients that form part of the diet have the potential to influence the body, and that in this respect there is little difference between food and medicine. This principle had been known and successfully practised by physicians for many generations before the advent of the modern polarised sciences of nutrition and medicine. In the words of the ancient Greek physician Hippocrates, 'Let food be thy medicine and medicine thy food.'

Until recently the substances in plants which were seen as being essential for their basic functioning, called primary metabolites, were the focus of attention for botanists. The secondary metabolites were considered to be useless, being regarded as potentially toxic waste products. Whilst the potential of plant toxins for use in medicine has always been recognised, the secondary metabolites are now being regarded in a new light. Not only are they seen to be important nutritional elements in feedingstuffs, but they have an important defensive role for the plant itself. With the benefit of hindsight, it is easy to see why species which have been bred with lower toxicity in order to increase their value as a food crop have not been as successful as they might have been. Not only are they more susceptible to disease, but they also lose their value as part of an holistic nutritional profile.

Toxicology

Chemical analysis of plants can determine their actual or supposed action on the chemistry of the body. However, for practical evaluation, there are other factors which must also be taken into consideration. For example, not all parts of some poisonous plants are toxic, and some are more toxic at certain times of year and even certain times of day. For instance, at nine o'clock in the morning, the opium poppy is reputed to contain four times as much morphine as it does at twelve noon. Also small amounts of some potentially toxic species can be beneficial for animals if ingested as part of an holistic nutritional profile, which means that a plant may be regarded as poisonous in some circumstances but not in others.

The time taken from eating a poisonous plant to the appearance of the first symptoms may vary greatly. For example, the effects of eating the leaves of yew and the roots of cowbane can be seen much more quickly than those produced by eating bracken and ragwort. Also the effect of some plants can vary greatly depending on the species of animal. This can be accounted for in some species simply as a result of the digestive process itself, which breaks down the poisonous element, but in others, complex chemical factors are involved. It is known that pigs will thrive on amounts of acorns which would be fatal in other species. Deer are reported to be able to feed on rhododendron leaves, which contain several toxic diterpenoids capable of causing rapid respiratory failure and death in sheep, goats and cattle. There are also variations within certain species: for example, some breeds of rabbit are not adversely affected by deadly nightshade whereas it causes death in others.

Traditionally plants have been classified according to their poisonous principles. There are a great many of these, including alkaloids, glycosides, saponins, nitrates, oxalates, tannins, photo-dynamic substances, minerals, phenols, volatile oils, etc. These are either synthesised by a chemical process within the plant itself, or concentrated by the plant from the soil. Many of these groups overlap chemically, and other classifications are possible, but the primary poisonous principles of most plants in Britain are alkaloids or glycosides.

Alkaloids

Alkaloids are present in many species of plants and are the dominant poisonous principle in high-risk toxic plants such as yew and hemlock. As well as being poisonous, alkaloids can also be used for medicinal purposes: they can be stimulants, depressives, narcotics, or painkillers. Alkaloids are the basis for many modern drugs, such as morphine, quinine, atropine and codeine. The alkaloid-containing plants are usually avoided by horses as they have a characteristic bitter taste, although some animals become addicted to them, even after showing symptoms of poisoning. Treatment of poisoned animals involves the use of drugs to counteract the effect of the alkaloid on the central nervous system. However, in those that do survive recovery is seldom complete.

Glycosides

Glycosides are a large group of organic substances, many of which are not poisonous. Those that are may be divided into four main categories which determine their toxicity, although some poisonous glycosides do not fit these groups. The groups are:

Cyanogenic

Cyanogenic plants are not toxic as such, but become so after they have been broken down by the digestive system, releasing the poisonous chemical, hydrocyanic acid (cyanide). Cyanogenic plants include those from the families Rosaceae, Leguminosae, and Gramineae. The flax plant is cyanogenic, which is why its seeds must be boiled before feeding to destroy its poisonous principle.

Goitrogenic

Most poisonous plants in this category are from the Cruciferae family such as cabbage and turnips. Plant goitrogens inhibit the uptake of iodine by the body, and poisoning is indicated by an increase in the size of the thyroid gland, which is recognised clinically as a goitre. Whereas goitres arising from iodine deficiencies in some hardwater areas may be treated by giving iodine, this treatment probably has no effect after poisoning by plant goitrogens, because the causative mechanism is different.

Cardiac

Cardiac glycosides have a direct action on the heart muscle, increasing its contractions whist slowing the rate. The other effects of these glycosides are gastro-enteritis and diarrhoea. In cases of poisoning, surgical elimination of the plant from the system is usually the only option. If lethal quantities of the substance are ingested and undisturbed, death occurs within 12–24 hours. The foxglove is the best known source of cardiac glycosides such as digitoxin, which has been used in medicine for many generations for the treatment of heart problems. Lily of the valley and hellebore *spp.* are other sources of cardiac glycosides.

Saponic

Saponic glycosides, or saponins, are distinguishable by their ability to form a lather (sapo means soap) and to emulsify oils. They are widely distributed and found in forage legumes such as lucerne, clover and many other plants. Saponins are more toxic to animals when injected than when eaten, although ingestion of large quantities can cause diarrhoea. Some are used medicinally as diuretics and others as expectorants. The saponin in liquorice root has similarities in action to the hormone cortisone, which is used in conventional drug therapy to treat inflammation.

Nitrates/nitrites

Nitrates are not very toxic in themselves but are converted by bacteria in the alimentary tract into nitrites, which are much more toxic. Nitrates are absorbed by plants from the soil and the rate of absorption can be increased by several factors, such as shade, the use of herbicides, and especially the use of nitrogenous fertilisers. Some foodstuffs, such as beet, turnips, mangles, rape, swedes and kale are more likely to accumulate high levels of nitrates than others, but accumulation in other plants can be significant.

Nitrites pass from the gastro-intestinal tract into the bloodstream, where they combine with elements in the blood to form a substance called methaemoglobin, which limits oxygen transportation. Symptoms of poisoning by nitrites, therefore, are those of oxygen deficiency, i.e. weakness, rapid weak pulse, a fall in blood pressure etc. Death from eating nitrate-rich feedingstuffs can occur within hours of ingestion, or more commonly it can take days for the symptoms of poisoning to appear. Ingestion of high levels of nitrogen have also been linked to infertility, abortion and vitamin imbalances.

Oxalates

Oxalates exist in many species of plants but are potentially more highly concentrated in certain types. Large variations exist in the amount of oxalates present in different species of plants at any one time, depending on the soil conditions, and climate. Differences also occur at various stages of growth; normally the toxin becomes more concentrated as the plant matures, particularly in the leaves.

The effect of eating the plant varies greatly, depending on the amount taken over a given period, and on the nutritional status of the animal, the amount of calcium in the diet etc. In cases of poisoning the following symptoms may be observed: rapid and laboured breathing, staggering, recumbency and depression. Some animals, including horses, can become adapted over a period of time to higher levels of oxalates in their diet, the greatest risk being when large amounts of oxalate-rich plants are consumed quickly. Hypocalcemia is produced, which is caused by the combination of the oxalates with calcium in the blood. On post-mortem of affected animals, various tissues and organs, notably the kidneys, contain deposits of calcium oxalate crystals.

Photosensitive agents

Photosensitive agents cause unpigmented or partially pigmented areas of the skin, such as the muzzle, to become hypersensitive to ultraviolet rays in sunlight, and this causes cell damage. These agents, the furocoumarins, are contained in several species of plants, notably St John's wort. Some of them do not require ingestion to produce hypersensitivity, as skin contact will also produce a reaction.

Primary photosensitivity by ingestion occurs when the furocoumarins are transported by the body unchanged to the surface of the skin. Secondary photosensitivity can also take place after the plant has been broken down by digestion, and the likelihood of this is increased if the alimentary capacity of the liver has been compromised. Therefore sensitivity to ultraviolet rays may be increased by secondary photosensitivity if liver damage has occurred through disease, hepatoxic drugs, agricultural chemicals etc.

Danger ratings

The plants in this booklet are divided into two basic groups which are represented by a symbol that appears alongside each entry. Qualified advice should be taken if there is the slightest doubt about the identity of plants that are suspected of being toxic.

Explanation of the symbols.

1.

High risk. Do not allow access.

2.

May be appropriate for ingestion on a regular basis depending on the overall nutritional profile together with the health status of the horse, but can be a hazard in some circumstances. If horses have been grazing for some time on pastures containing such plants, there is probably little to be concerned about providing the horses are healthy. An eye should always be kept on the quantity of these plants in relation to other species and advice taken if they (or any other plants) increase dramatically. Qualified advice should be taken if there is the slightest doubt. Information is available from the Veterinary Poisons Information Unit or the British Association of Holistic Nutrition and Medicine (see p. 69).

Acorns (from *Quercus* spp.)
See Oak.

Alder buckthorn (*Frangula alnus*)
A deciduous non-spiny shrub growing to about 3 m in height. It is a native of Britain although absent from Scotland, and likes calcareous soils, preferring damp woods, scrub, bogs and fenland. A preparation made from the bark of alder buckthorn is used medicinally as a mild laxative.

Poisonous principles and symptoms
The plant contains glycosides which produce purgative anthraquinones. Symptoms of poisoning may include diarrhoea, cramps, slight fever. Reported cases of poisoning in equines are rare.

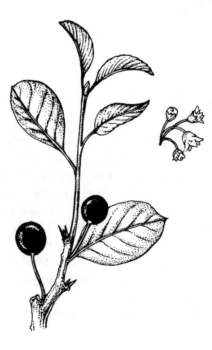

Black bryony (*Tamus communis*)

A climbing plant preferring the edges of woods, scrub and hedges. Common throughout southern England, the Midlands and Wales, absent from Scotland.

Poisonous principles and symptoms

Very little is known about its poisonous principle, but it is thought to be a glycoside. Symptoms may include decreased appetite with severe abdominal pains, high temperature and profuse sweating. Some reported cases of fatal equine poisoning.

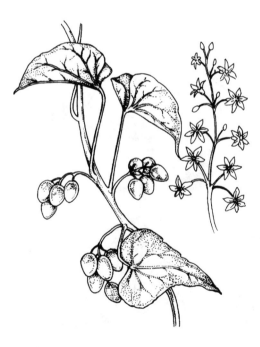

Black nightshade (*Solanum nigrum*)

An erect branched annual (occasionally biennial) plant, measuring from under 10 cm up to 60 cm, which is a highly successful and troublesome weed in cultivated land.

Poisonous principles and symptoms

The plant, particularly the berries, contains toxic alkaloids, nitrates and nitrites. Symptoms of poisoning may include severe abdominal pain, staggering and depression. The plant varies in toxicity according to several factors such as climate, season and soil type. This may account for conflicting reports concerning its toxicity. Few reports of poisoning in equines.

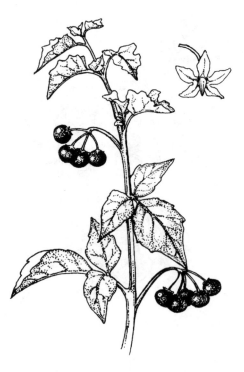

Box **17**

Box (*Buxus sempervirens*)

A native evergreen shrub or tree, limited to southern England and found on chalk or limestone and in woods and scrubland. Box is cultivated as a garden hedging plant.

Poisonous principles and symptoms

All parts of the plant are poisonous, but it is usually avoided by animals presumably because of its unpleasant taste. it contains a substance called buxine which is composed of a complex group of steroidal alkaloids. Symptoms of poisoning include diarrhoea, incoordination, convulsions and coma. Respiratory failure is the usual cause of death. Poisoning has been reported in horses, usually after gaining access to gardens containing the plant or access to clippings.

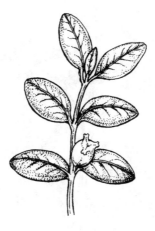

Bracken (*Pteridium aquilinum*)

A fern plant measuring up to two metres in height and common in woodland areas of Great Britain. It prefers acid soil and has a creeping underground root system, from which leaves sprout in the spring, dying down again in the autumn.

Poisonous principles and symptoms

Bracken is carcinogenic as well as containing an enzyme, thyaminase, which leads to thiamine (vitamin B1) deficiency. Symptoms of thiamine deficiency include incoordination, pronounced heartbeat after mild exercise, and muscle tremors. If untreated (intravenous administration of thiamine) this is followed by convulsions and death. The symptoms gave rise to the old name of 'bracken staggers'. Bracken is a common cause of serious or fatal poisoning in horses.

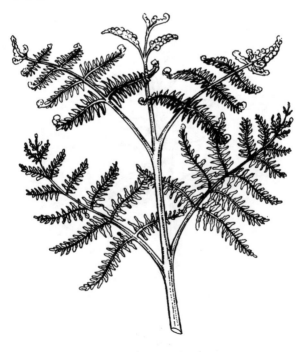

Broom (*Cytisus scoparius*)

A shrub that is common in dry hilly areas throughout Britain, western Europe and Scandinavia. Used in herbal medicine, it has cardio-active and diuretic properties, and should only be used medicinally by appropriately qualified and experienced practitioners. Broom tops are a traditional anthelmintic.

Poisonous principles and symptoms

The plant contains alkaloids which can depress the heart and nervous system and paralyse the motor nerve endings. No reported cases of poisoning in equines, probably due to the fact that the small leaves and wiry stems make it unattractive to them.

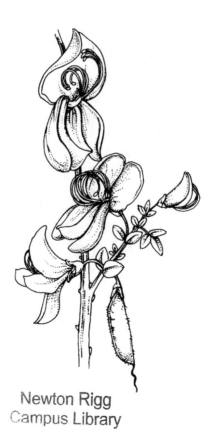

Buckthorn (*Rhamnus cathartica*)

A thorny deciduous shrub reaching 4–6 m in height. It prefers calcareous soils and is a native of Britain. Buckthorn can be used medicinally as a laxative. Other common names – Purging buckthorn, Common buckthorn.

Poisonous principles and symptoms

See Alder Buckthorn.

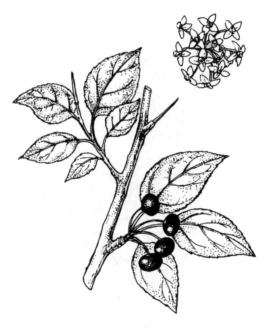

Buckwheat (*Fagopyrum esculentum*)

Buckwheat is native to Central Asia and is cultivated on a small scale in Britain and also in other parts of the world. In America it is the source of buckwheat flour which is used to make pancakes. It is used in herbal medicine for conditions involving the circulatory system. It occurs wild occasionally on waste ground.

Poisonous principles and symptoms

A pigment called fagopyrin is thought to be the poisonous principle of the plant but relatively little is known about its chemical profile in this respect. The dehusked seeds are thought to be harmless and commonly used in animal feeds; however, animals which have ingested large quantities of the fresh or dried plant have developed photosensitivity to sunlight. Symptoms include reddening of the skin which may develop lesions, nervousness, agitation, and emaciation.

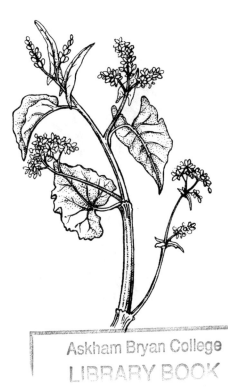

Buttercup (*Ranunculus acris*)

A hairy perennial plant widespread throughout Britain in pastures and meadows, preferring alkaline soils. Other common names – Meadow buttercup, Field buttercup, Tall buttercup.

Poisonous principles and symptoms

Meadow buttercup, in common with other plants of the same family, such as greater spearwort (*Ranunculus lingua*), contains a toxic compound called protoanemonin. In large quantities this compound causes salivation, together with inflammation of the mouth and abdominal pain with convulsions usually preceding death. However, very few cases of poisoning involving plants of the *Ranunculus* family have been reported. Even so the plants must be regarded as a potential risk. Protoanemonin is an unstable compound which is changed to a non-toxic substance when the plant is dried. This means that hay containing buttercups (or any other member of the same family) is safe to feed to horses.

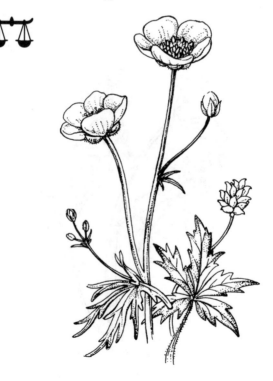

Celandine, greater (*Chelidonium majus*)

An erect branched plant reaching 60 cm in height, with smooth or slightly hairy stems. Preferring banks and hedgerows, and found in most parts of Britain except Scotland. Traditionally used in the external treatment of warts, and internally for liver, lung, gastro-intestinal problems, and rheumatism. Other common names – Celandine poppy, Wart wort.

Poisonous principles and symptoms

The plant contains many potentially toxic alkaloids such as chelidonine. Symptoms of poisoning may include excessive salivation and urination, thirst, drowsiness, cessation of bowel movement, and staggering gait. Post-mortem findings may include gastro-intestinal irritation. Poisoning is comparatively rare owing to the fact that the plant is probably normally unattractive, having a feotid smell and acid taste.

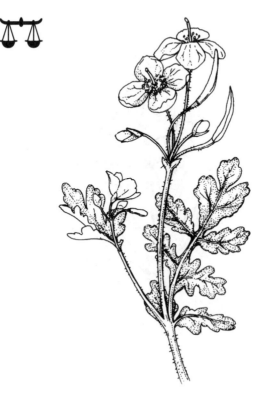

Charlock (*Sinapis arvensis*)

An annual weed of arable land preferring calcareous and heavy soils. Charlock has been controlled by selective weedkillers and is therefore less common today than it once was. It has bright yellow flowers which are present for most of the summer and the seeds are capable of remaining dormant in the ground for a number of years. The seeds of the plant have been used in herbal medicine for digestive problems.

Poisonous principles and symptoms

The seeds of charlock are poisonous, containing a volatile mustard oil, allyl isothiocyanate. Symptoms of poisoning include acute gastroenteritis, frothing at the mouth, grunting and diarrhoea. Large amounts can cause bloat, breathing difficulty, bulging eyes and shuffling gait. Death is caused by asphyxia in 1–2 hours. Cases of poisoning in horses have been reported.

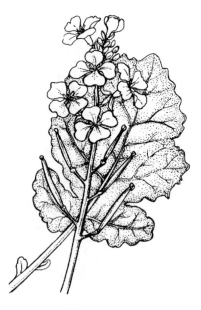

Chickweed (*Stellaria media*)

One of the commonest weeds with world-wide distribution. Found in gardens, fields, waste ground, etc. Used in homoeopathy for the treatment of rheumatism, arthritis and bronchitis.

Poisonous principles and symptoms

Chickweed contains saponins which can cause digestive upsets and diarrhoea, but has only very rarely been associated with poisoning. It is only likely to be consumed in quantity in times of severe grass shortage.

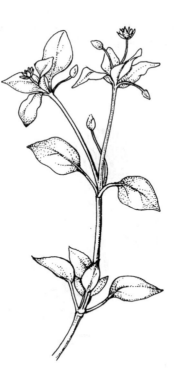

Clover (Trifolium spp.)

Many types of clover are found in Britain. These include red clover (Trifolium *pratense*), white clover (Trifolium *repens* – illustrated), subterranean clover (Trifolium *subterraneum*), and alsike clover (Trifolium *hybridum*), together with many cultivated varieties which are grown for grazing or hay or to be ploughed into the ground to increase nitrogen in the soil.

Poisonous principles and symptoms

Clovers may contain oestrogens, cyanogenic glycosides, goitrogens, nitrates and other substances which may cause health problems in horses. These can be associated with laminitis, blood coagulation disorders and photosensitivity. There are also diseases which may be caused by fungi which infect clover. Whilst clover has caused poisoning in horses, due to agricultural methods and possibly the strains of the plant available, there are few reported cases in Britain.

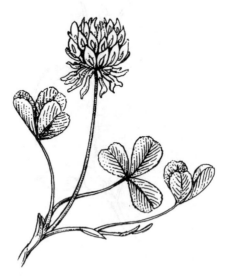

Columbine (*Aquilegia vulgaris*)

A perennial plant reaching 30–60 cm. A native of Britain, preferring chalk soils and found on shady slopes and in woodland. Columbine is found only locally in Britain although many other hybrids and species are cultivated in gardens.

Poisonous principles and symptoms

Columbine contains toxic alkaloids which in theory could cause asphyxia and respiratory failure, although there are no reported cases of poisoning in horses.

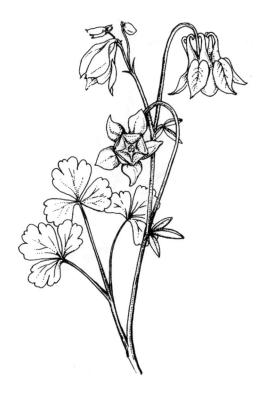

Corncockle (*Agrostemma githago*)

An annual plant reaching 30–100 cm in height. The corncockle is not native to Britain but was formerly a common weed in cereal crops, as it still is in other parts of the world. The leaves are covered in white hairs which gives the plant a greyish appearance and the single flowers are pink.

Poisonous principles and symptoms

The corncockle contains colloidal glycosides which have the properties of saponin. Symptoms of poisoning include salivation, gastro-intestinal disturbance and paralysis. Frothy diarrhoea has also been observed. Saponin-containing plants have a bitter taste and are not readily eaten, but there are reports of the corncockle causing poisoning in horses.

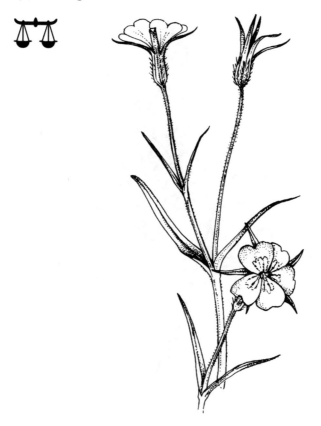

Cowbane (*Cicuta virosa*)

An erect perennial plant reaching 30–130 cm high, preferring damp locations such as shallow water, ditches and marshes. It is found in localised areas of Britain such as East Anglia, some parts of the Midlands, Scotland and Ireland.

Poisonous principles and symptoms

The roots of the cowbane contain a concentrated higher alcohol known as cicutoxin which is a convulsive poison, small quantities being sufficient to kill a horse. Symptoms may include salivation, dilated pupils, spasmodic convulsions, abdominal pain. There is not normally diarrhoea. The leaves and stems are also poisonous but to a lesser degree than the roots. The greatest risk of poisoning is when the roots are exposed after ditching.

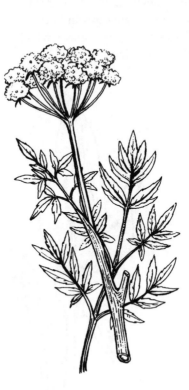

Cuckoo pint (*Arum maculatum*)

A plant generally widely distributed in Great Britain but less common in northern parts. It prefers a shady situation such as woods and hedge banks and is a persistent weed in some gardens. It is also called lords and ladies which is related particularly to the fruiting stage. Other common name: Arum lily.

Poisonous principles and symptoms

The juice of the plant is an acute irritant when applied to the skin or ingested. The nature of the toxic principle is not certain but it is thought to be a saponin which is present in all parts of the plant. Symptoms include salivation, swelling of the neck, incoordination, followed by collapse and death. Poisoning is rare presumably because of the pungent taste of the plant. Arum poisoning was suspected in seven separate cases in horses in Britain over a period of five years. All were pregnant mares which subsequently aborted and five of the animals died.

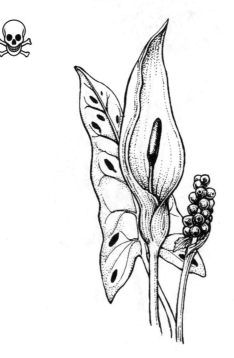

Darnel (Lolium temulentum)

An erect annual grass which reaches a height of about 1 metre. Darnel is the only British grass which is potentially harmful and although it used to be a common weed in cereal crops, it is now rare. There are many accounts from ancient times of people and animals being poisoned by eating food made with flour contaminated with darnel seeds.

Poisonous principles and symptoms

Although its poisonous principle is not clear, it is thought to be associated with alkaloids. Fungi, either in or on the leaves, have also been associated with various toxins. Symptoms of alkaloid poisoning may include excessive salivation (or absence), dilation of pupils, abdominal pain, diarrhoea, incoordination and liver dysfunction. Toxicity studies of darnel have produced inconsistent conclusions, for example in some instances contaminated feed appears to have no ill effects.

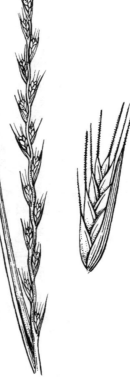

Deadly nightshade (*Atropa belladonna*)

A smooth slightly hairy perennial, reaching about 1.5 m high, preferring calcareous soils. It is found in woodland and on waste and stoney ground in central Europe and southern Britain. The plant is rich in alkaloids and can be used medicinally to reduce spasm in the gut wall and for some conditions of the urinary tract. It can also be used to reduce salivation and perspiration. A few drops in the eye dilates the pupil which facilitates examination.

Poisonous principles and symptoms

Deadly nightshade contains various alkaloids and as its name suggests it is highly toxic. Symptoms of poisoning may include dilated pupils, inflamed mucus membranes, nervous excitement and inability to stand. The plant is seldom eaten by horses, presumably because of its unpleasant taste.

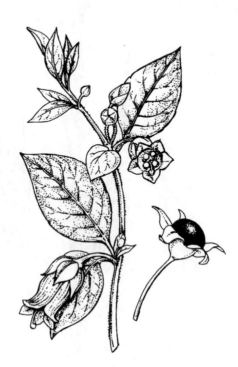

Foxglove (*Digitalis purpurea*)

An erect biennial plant reaching 150 cm in height, found growing wild and in gardens throughout Europe. It has red/purple (occasionally white) helmet-shaped flowers. The leaves of the foxglove are the source of digitalis which is used medicinally for heart and kidney problems.

Poisonous principles and symptoms

The foxglove contains the cardiac glycosides digitoxin, digitalin, digitonin, digitalosmin, gitoxin and gitalonin. Signs of poisoning include diarrhoea, abdominal pain, irregular pulse, tremors and convulsions. Foxglove is not usually eaten, but animals can develop a craving for it once ingested. It does not lose its toxicity when dried and hay containing foxglove may present a higher risk than the growing plant.

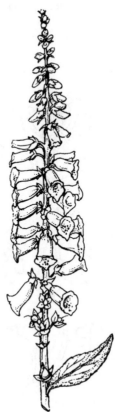

Ground ivy (*Glechoma hederacea*)

A creeping native plant of Britain growing to about 20 cm tall. It smells rather unpleasant and prefers grassland, woodland edges, waste ground and damp woods. Used in herbal medicine as a blood cleanser, tonic and diuretic, also to treat kidney stones and gastritis. The leaves are said to reduce inflammation.

Poisonous principles and symptoms

Ground ivy contains oils and a bitter substance which are not clearly characterised. There appears to be no reported cases of poisoning in Britain; however, there are reports of illness and death associated with the plant amongst horses in eastern Europe. Symptoms include accelerated weak pulse, respiratory distress, elevated temperature and dizziness. Post-mortem examination may reveal enlargement of the spleen, dilation of the caecum and gastroenteritis.

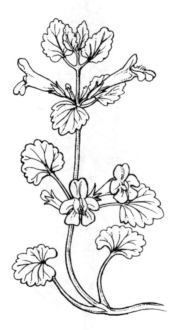

Hellebore (*Helleborus spp.*)

There are several species of hellebores and there is often confusion which arises over the use of their common names. The species native to Britain are *Helleborus viridis* and *Helleborus foetidus* (illustrated) which are restricted to calcareous soils and are local in distribution. There are also cultivated hybrids grown in gardens throughout the country. The hellebore has been used in medicine as a purgative, as a local anaesthetic, as an abortive and as an antiparasitic.

Poisonous principles and symptoms

Hellebores contain glycosides under various names, including helliborin and others. Symptoms of poisoning may include loss of coat condition, tremors, respiratory problems, irregular pulse, abdominal pain, diarrhoea, excessive urination. There are few reported cases of poisoning in horses.

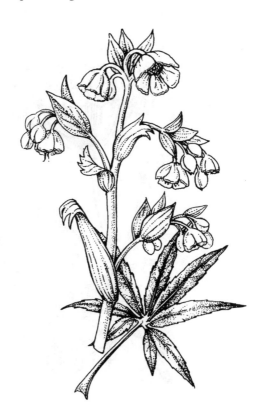

Hemlock (*Conium maculatum*)

An erect branched biennial plant reaching 2 m or more in height. Found growing in ditches, on roadsides and waste ground; common in Europe except western and central Scotland, also found in Asia. Hemlock was formerly used in herbal medicine to treat neurological disorders, as a sedative and anaesthetic. The plant is highly toxic and was used by the Ancient Greeks as a form of execution. Socrates was killed by it. It is easily confused with other umbellifers, except for its size and the prominent purple spotting on the stem.

Poisonous principles and symptoms

Hemlock contains a group of poisonous alkaloids which are found in highest concentration in parts other than the root. Symptoms of poisoning include paralysis and convulsions. Death occurs through respiratory paralysis. Poisoning has been reported in horses.

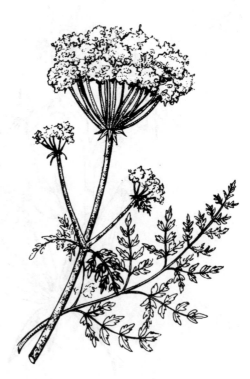

Hemlock water-dropwort (*Oenanthe crocata*)

An erect perennial plant growing to about 50–150 cm high, preferring damp places and calcareous soils. Found throughout Britain. The rootstock is composed of five or more fleshy, pale yellow or white finger-like tubers, hence its common name 'dead men's fingers'.

Poisonous principles and symptoms

The plant contains a concentrated higher alcohol which is a convulsant poison not affected either by drying or storage. The roots are the most toxic part of the plant and very small amounts can cause death. The greatest concentration of the toxins in the plant is during the winter and it is most troublesome during ditching operations which expose the roots at that time of year. Symptoms of poisoning include salivation, dilated pupils, convulsions and death, which usually rapidly follows ingestion of the plant.

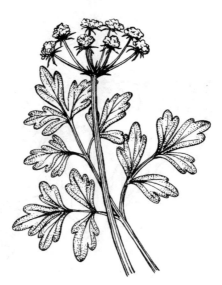

Hemp nettle (*Galeopsis ladanum*)

Otherwise known as broad-leaved hemp nettle, the hemp nettle is not native to the British Isles but has been introduced. It is found mainly on waste land. It has a softly hairy stem and small lilac flowers which appear in July to September.

Poisonous principles and symptoms

Hemp nettle is said to have caused poisoning of horses in Europe but there have been no recent documented reports. The poisonous principle of the plant is not clear. Affected animals appear weak and refuse their feed and water and display muscle tremors. Post-mortem examinations have shown haemorrhagic inflammation of the stomach and small intestine.

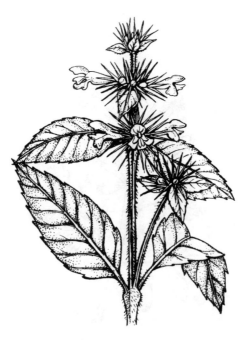

Henbane (*Hyoscyamus niger*)

An annual or biennial plant preferring waste ground, old buildings, coastal sand or shingle. Found in Europe, Asia, and north Africa. Once cultivated for use in medicine as a sedative and painkiller.

Poisonous principles and symptoms

Henbane contains tropane alkaloids and all parts of the plant, particularly the roots, are poisonous. Symptoms may include restlessness, convulsions, rapid heartbeat, dilated pupils and dry mouth. The plant has a disagreeable odour which makes it unattractive to animals in normal circumstances. No reports of equine poisoning with henbane have been reported in Britain since the early twentieth century.

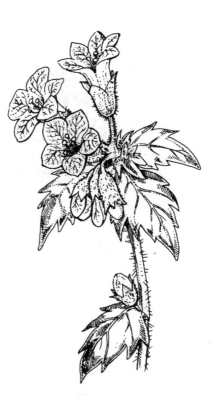

Herb Paris (*Paris quadrifolia*)

A hairless perennial plant that is native to Britain but only found locally in western areas. It grows to about 40 cm tall, preferring damp calcareous soil and found, usually in woodland, in most of Europe and Asia. Herb Paris is used in homoeopathy to treat problems associated with the nervous system.

Poisonous principles and symptoms

There is little published information on the plant that is of any value, mainly because it is confusing. The toxins are thought to be saponins or glycosides. Reports of poisoning include symptoms such as excitability, nervous twitching, and increased pulse. Painful urination and bowel movements, together with dilated pupils, have also been observed later. The plant is unpalatable in normal circumstances and poisoning in horses is rare.

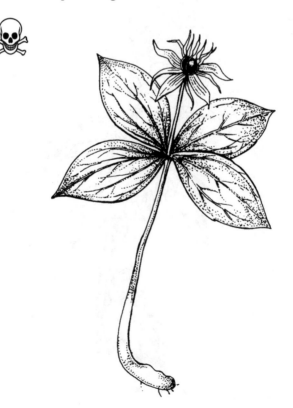

Horse radish (*Armoracia rusticana*)

A robust perennial plant reaching 1.5 m tall with a thick fleshy root. It was introduced to Britain from Western Asia and can be found in waste ground, fields, beside watercourses and cultivated for human consumption. It is used medicinally for respiratory and urinary problems and as a poultice for rheumatism and bronchitis.

Poisonous principles and symptoms

Horse radish contains a substance called sinigrin, which is a potent irritant, along with other toxins. Poisoning is rare presumably because of the pungent taste of the plant but there have been reports in Britain of poisoning in horses. In one case six ponies were found dead after breaking into an orchard and gorging themselves on the leaves and flowering stems of the plant. There was evidence of violent struggling before death and post-mortem examination revealed acute inflammation of the stomach.

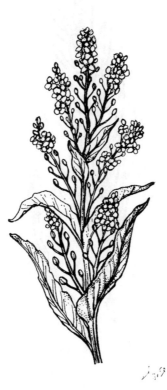

Horsetail (Equisetum spp.)

A plant with vegetative stems up to 80 cm tall. Preferring damp grassy sites and found throughout Europe, Asia and North America. There are around ten species that occur in Britain, the common horsetail (Equisetum arvense – illustrated) and the marsh horsetail (Equisetum palustre) being the most common. Used in traditional medicine to treat kidney and bladder disorders, also for eczema and arthritis.

Poisonous principles and symptoms

Horsetail contains an enzyme called thiaminase which is antagonistic to thiamine (vitamin B1). See Bracken. Significant intake can lead to kidney damage.

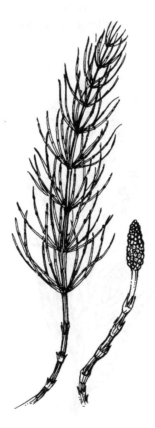

Iris (Iris *pseudacorus*/*foetidissima*)

There are two types of iris commonly found in Britain, the yellow flag (Iris *pseudacorus*) and the stinking iris (Iris *foetidissima* – illustated). The yellow flag is found in marshes and wet ground and the stinking iris in hedgerows, woodland, and on sea cliffs.

Poisonous principles and symptoms

All parts of both species are poisonous, especially the rhizomes. The poisonous principle is not clear but the plants contain resin, a glycoside, myristic acid and an acrid compound. Symptoms of poisoning include elevation of temperature, intestinal disturbance with diarrhoea and sometimes bleeding. Poisoning of horses has been reported with recovery in a few days.

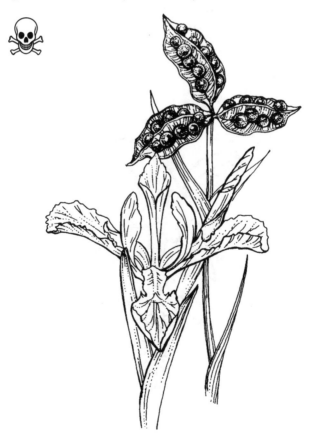

Laburnum (*Laburnum anagyroides*)

A tree growing 7–9 m high and commonly found as an ornamental species in gardens throughout the country. It does not grow wild in Britain, except as an escape from cultivation. The bright yellow flowers are similar to those of the pea and the seed pods are often seen hanging on the tree throughout the winter. Other common names – Golden chain, Golden rain.

Poisonous principles and symptoms

Laburnum contains an alkaloid called cysticine which is found in all parts of the tree, particularly the bark and seeds. Symptoms of poisoning may include abdominal pain, elevated temperature, tremors, unsteady gait and convulsions. Fatal poisoning in horses has been reported, mostly involving high consumption of seeds and pods eaten from trees to which they had been tied.

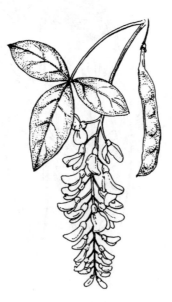

Larkspur (*Consolida ajacis*)

Although not a native species, there is considerable variation of size and form of larkspur (also known as delphinium) that are cultivated throughout Britain. The elongated spur on the (usually, but not always) blue flowers is a distinguishing feature.

Poisonous principles and symptoms

All species of *Consolida* (*Delphinium*) are poisonous, containing alkaloids such as delphinine and ajacine. The highest concentration is in young plants and seeds. Symptoms of poisoning may include agitation, breathing difficulties, incoordination, abdominal pain, muscular spasms and difficulty in standing. Animals are unlikely to ingest the plant unless they have access to gardens or garden rubbish containing it. Few reported cases of poisoning in horses.

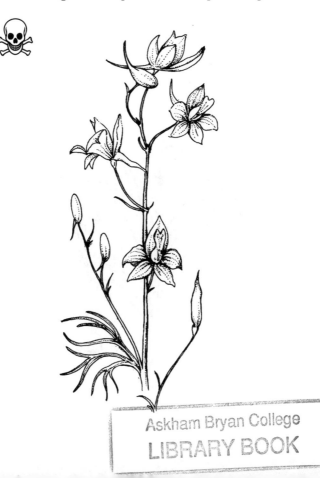

Lily of the valley (*Convallaria majalis*)

A small perennial plant with white bell-shaped flowers which appear in the spring. It is native to Britain and widely cultivated. The plant is used in medicine to treat conditions of the heart, particularly those involving heart muscle and heart-related fluid retention.

Poisonous principles and symptoms

There is some confusion about the poisonous principle. The lily of the valley contains the glycosides convallerin, convallomarin and convallotoxin, convallotoxin being strongly associated with the toxic nature of the plant. Symptoms of poisoning may include gastro-intestinal disturbance, irregular pulse, excess salivation and dilated pupils. There are few reported cases of fatal poisoning in horses.

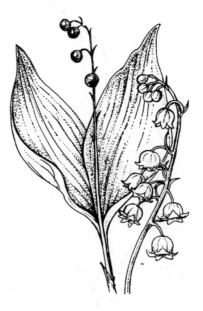

Linseed (*Linum usitatissimum*)

The seed of the flax plant, cultivated in Britain for its oil and also for the fibrous stem of the plant. It contains useful protein and valuable oils and can be used as a conditioner and mild laxative.

Poisonous principles and symptoms

Linseed contains the cyanogenic glycoside linamarin, which after digestion produces the poison hydrocyanic acid. This prevents utilisation of oxygen in the body and death is caused by oxygen starvation to the brain. The poisonous principle of the plant is destroyed by heat and linseed must be thoroughly cooked before being given to horses.

Symptoms of poisoning may include salivation, staggering, dilated pupils, rapid pulse, gasping, inability to stand and convulsions. In some cases death can be instantaneous and no symptoms are seen.

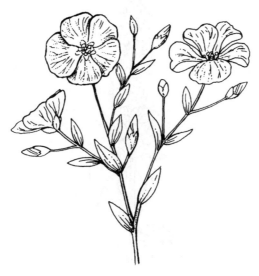

Lupin (Lupinus spp.)

Lupins are perennial plants reaching 1 m high. Although not a native species, many varieties are cultivated throughout Britain, being mainly the species L. *polyphyllus*. These are mostly found in gardens, but sometimes grow wild, having been thrown out in garden rubbish. Although the lupin is listed as a poison, in some parts of the world some varieties are grown for forage.

Poisonous principles and symptoms

The so-called 'bitter' varieties contain several toxic alkaloids. A substance called biochanin is also present in some species, which has the potential to cause reproductive disorders. Symptoms of alkaloid poisoning include staggering, inability to stand and convulsions. Risk of poisoning is low as the 'bitter' varieties are probably unpalatable, and horses rarely have access to the plant unless it is contained in discarded garden waste.

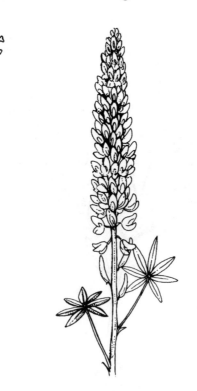

Marsh marigold (*Caltha palustris*)

Common in marshes and wet areas throughout Britain, often forming luxurious growth in shaded areas. Growing to about 30 cm high and bearing yellow flowers in early summer. The form of the plant may be variable. The plant is not related to other marigolds which are members of the Compositae family.

Poisonous principles and symptoms

In common with other plants of the Ranunculaceae family, the marsh marigold contains various toxins including, notably, an irritant substance called protoanemonin. The plant has an acrid taste and cases of poisoning are rare; however, animals have been known to develop a taste for the plant even though other food is available. Symptoms of poisoning are not well documented but they would probably include those seen in other cases of protoanemonin poisoning, for example salivation, abdominal pain and inflammation of the mouth.

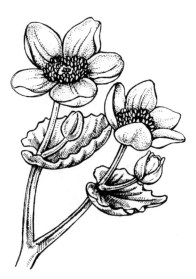

Meadow saffron (*Colchicum autumnale*)

A hairless perennial plant growing to about 25 cm tall and found in damp meadows in most of Europe. In Britain it is mainly found in central England. Meadow saffron is used medicinally in the homoeopathic treatment of rheumatism and circulatory problems. It is is also being investigated as a possible treatment for cancer. Other common names – Autumn crocus, Naked ladies.

Poisonous principles and symptoms

The plant contains a number of toxic alkaloids, of which colchicine is the most toxic. The alkaloids are particularly concentrated in the corm and seeds, but all parts of the plant are poisonous. Colchicine affects the nervous system, and symptoms of poisoning may include abdominal pain, salivation, severe diarrhoea, incoordination and collapse. Death may occur through circulatory or respiratory dysfunction. Few reports of poisoning in Britain but these have included horses.

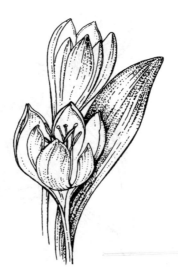

Melilot (*Melilotus spp.*)

There are three types of melilot that have become naturalised in Britain and commonly found in fields and waste ground, especially in the south of England. These are the common or ribbed melilot (*Melilotus officinalis*), the white melilot (*Melilotus albus* – illustrated) and the tall melilot (*Melilotus altissimus*). All three types are usually biennials and are similar in appearance. Also known as sweet clover. Used in herbal medicine to treat varicose veins and piles, and in homoeopathy for nosebleeds.

Poisonous principles and symptoms

Melilots are safe for grazing, but when incorporated into hay certain constituents of the plants called coumarins may be converted into a substance which impairs blood clotting. Where large quantities have been ingested, fatal haemorrhaging has occurred within a short time, with subcutaneous haemorrhaging, pale mucous membrane, weakness and rapid heartbeat occurring immediately prior to death. This principle has been made use of in rodenticides. Owing to the scarcity of the plant in pastures it is unlikely to be a problem in most hay grown in Great Britain. There are isolated cases of poisoning in old literature but no recent reports.

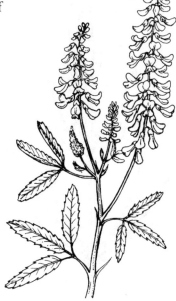

Mercury (*Mercurialis* spp.)

Mercurialis perennis, or dog's mercury (illustrated), grows throughout Britain, commonly in woodland. It grows from long creeping rhizomes and has a branched stem about 40 cm tall. The other common species is *Mercurialis annua* which is probably not a native species but which is widely estabished in southern England. It has erect branched stems reaching about 10–50 cm high, growing on waste land and as a garden weed.

Poisonous principles and symptoms

Both species are poisonous but the actual poisonous principles have not been studied in detail. They are thought to be associated with, amongst other things, saponins and a volatile oil. Although the plant has an unpleasant taste and poisoning is rare, animals will take the plant when other food is scarce and have been known to develop a taste for it. Symptoms include gastrointestinal upset, jaundice of oral and genital mucous membrane and eyes, salivation, diarrhoea, weakness, lethargy, blood-stained urine and coma which may precede death.

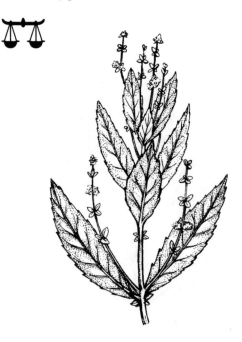

Monk's hood (*Aconitum napellus*)

A perennial plant growing to around 100 cm high, a rare plant preferring high altitude woodland, damp woods and riverbanks. Monk's hood is used in conventional medicine as a local anaesthetic and in homoeopathy for the treatment of fevers and in some heart conditions. The plant is also used in Traditional Chinese Medicine for the treatment of heart disease.

Poisonous principles and symptoms

Monk's hood is reputed to be Britain's most poisonous plant. It contains extremely toxic alkaloids such as aconitine and other similar types. Symptoms of poisoning may include, at first, a stimulatory effect on the respiration and circulation, followed by a depression with slow laboured breathing and low pulse. Large amounts usually produce sudden death from asphyxia and circulatory collapse. Early reports of poisoning include horses, but the risk is currently small as the plant is comparatively rare.

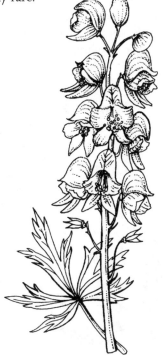

Oak (*Quercus spp.*)

A native tree found in most parts of England. Growing in woodland, parkland and hedges, it may live to be many hundreds of years old. Oak bark or 'tanner's bark' used to be used for tanning leather and an extract from the tree can be used medicinally for the treatment of diarrhoea. Powdered nut galls can be used as an astringent in the treatment of surface tissue where a limited circulatory effect is required.

Poisonous principles and symptoms

The oak contains tannins which can be highly toxic, but information on the potential of the tree to poison animals often appears to be contradictory. Whilst there are reports of horses eating acorns with apparently little ill effect (they have also been given as a highly nutritious winter feed), there is no doubt that fatalities have occurred after ingestion of these and other parts of the tree. Reports are more common in the autumn when acorns are more abundant. Symptoms of poisoning may include constipation and blood-stained faeces, refusal to drink, weakness and staggering, irregular slow heart beat, pale mucus membrane and watery eyes. The kidneys can be damaged in extreme cases.

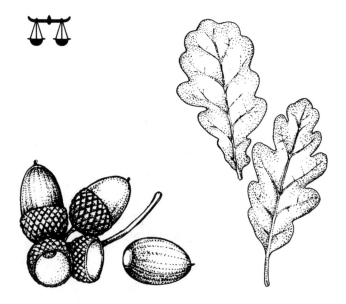

Pimpernel (*Anagallis arvensis*)

A small annual or perennial plant reaching about 10 cm high. Preferring cultivated ground and waste land and found almost world-wide, the plant is used medicinally in the homoeopathic treatment of skin and liver problems. Other common names – Scarlet pimpernel, Shepherd's weather glass.

Poisonous principles and symptoms

Pimpernel has long been regarded as poisonous although its poisonous principle is uncertain. There are conflicting reports of its toxicity which may be due in part to the fact that, in common with many poisonous plants, the severity of its effects may vary considerably between individual animals. Pimpernel contains both glycosidal saponins and an acrid volatile oil and symptoms of poisoning may include gastro-intestinal problems, staggering, incoordination, difficult breathing, and in the final stages coma and a rapid drop in body temperature.

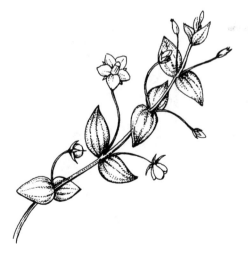

Poppy (*Papaver somniferum*)

A sturdy annual plant reaching 1.5 m high, preferring waste ground, also cultivated. Found in south-east Europe and western Asia, poppies are not native to Britain but may be occasionally found as relics of a former cultivation. The plant is commonly confused with the field poppy (*Papaver rhoeas*), which although not commonly regarded as poisonous, contains potentially toxic alkaloids. *Papaver somniferum* is the source of opium, which was once describe as 'the sheet anchor of the veterinarian'. The unripe seeds of the opium poppy are used in the manufacture of morphine and codeine, and tincture of opium produces laudanum. Other names – White poppy, Opium poppy.

Poisonous principles and symptoms

The plant contains a crude resin, opium, which is present in the whole plant, especially the seed pods. Symptoms may include restlessness, excessive salivation, increased respiration, reduction in body temperature, and narcosis.

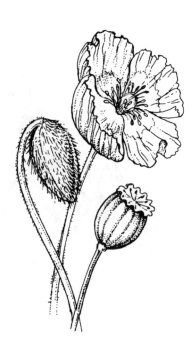

Potato (*Solanum tuberosum*)

The white underground tubers of the potato are widely cultivated for human consumption and have also been used as a horse food.

Poisonous principles and symptoms

The stems, leaves, flowers, and fruits (haulms) contain the glycoside, solanine, and other toxic substances. Symptoms may include gastro-intestinal problems, weak pulse, circulatory failure, incoordination, restlessness and convulsions. Coma and death may follow. Fatalities in horses have been reported. The related tomato plant may be similarly toxic.

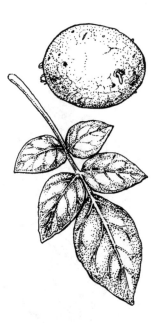

Privet (Ligustrum spp.)

Common privet (Ligustrum vulgare – illustrated) is a deciduous native shrub of Britain, preferring calcareous soil. It can reach a height of 5 m. Various types of privet, some of which are evergreen, are cultivated as garden shrubs, or as ornamental hedging plants.

Poisonous principles and symptoms

The poisonous principle of privet is not fully understood, but thought to be associated with the the glycoside, ligustrine. The berries are normally thought of as being toxic, but all arial parts of the plant have caused poisoning. Symptoms may include stagger-ing, intestinal disruption, paralysis, rapid pulse, congested mucous membrane and dilated pupils. Fatal cases of poisoning have been reported in horses, death occurring from 4–48 hours after ingestion of the plant. Most cases involve garden hedges or hedge trimmings.

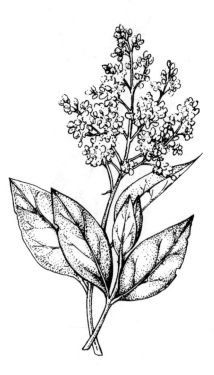

Ragwort (*Senecio jacobaea*)

A (usually) biennial plant, abundant in Britain, reaching 30–100 cm high, preferring waste-land, beside roads and in pastures. It has bright yellow flowers on erect stems and jagged lobed leaves, hence its name. Ragwort was designated as an injurious weed in the Weeds Act 1959. Under the Act a landowner can be required to prevent the plant from spreading, and failure to do so within a specified time renders him liable to prosecution.

Poisonous principles and symptoms

These are linked to the pyrrolizidine alkaloids, the most toxic of which are cyclic diesters. Symptoms may not appear until animals have been ingesting the plant for several weeks or months, although they can appear immediately. They include digestive disturbance, abdominal pain and diarrhoea, restlessness, incoordination and paralysis. There appears to be no correlation between the severity of the symptoms and the length of time the plant has been consumed by the animal. The name 'sleepy staggers' has been given to this condition in horses and many fatalities have been recorded. The plant does not lose its poisonous principle after dying and storage and contaminated hay has caused many problems. The plant should be sought out, uprooted and burnt. Fortunately the rooting system is shallow.

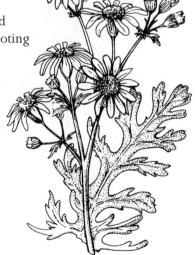

Rhododendron (*Rhododendron ponticum*)

An evergreen shrub reaching 3 m high, common in Britain, being found in woodland and cultivated in gardens and parks. The flowers are large and purple in colour, although many colours are seen in cultivated varieties.

Poisonous principles and symptoms

The leaves, pollen, flowers and nectar contain several toxic diterpenoids and the shrub has been recognised as a poison since ancient times. In 400 BC Xenophon reported poisoning of Greek soldiers from honey made by bees from wild rhododendrons (poisoning by honey from the plant in subsequent cultures is virtually unknown because of better apiary management). Symptoms of poisoning may include abdominal pain, salivation, diarrhoea, constipation, staggering, trembling, weak pulse, slow irregular breathing and collapse. The risk is normally associated with animals gaining access to woodland or gardens containing the shrub.

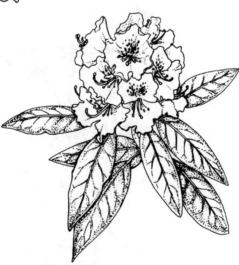

Rush (*Juncus spp.*)

Rushes are erect plants with long, stiff, narrow leaves. There are several species occurring in Britain (the flower of the compact rush (*Juncus conglomeratus*) is illustrated), growing mainly in marshy and wet areas, including poorly drained agricultural areas such as pastureland.

Poisonous principles and symptoms

There is little scientific information available on the poisonous principle, which is believed to be cyanide in the form of cyanogenic glycosides. The amount of toxins in the plant appears to fluctuate at different times of the year. Reports of poisoning are inconsistent and there is little known about the effects of eating the plant in Britain. In other countries animals that have been poisoned with rush have died suddenly as a result of oxygen starvation of the central nervous system, which is consistent with cyanide poisoning.

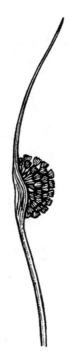

St John's wort (Hypericum perforatum)

An erect hairless plant usually 30–50 cm high (but can reach 1 m), preferring rocky slopes, dry grassland, meadows and open woods. Common in Britain and other parts of the world; rare in Scotland. Used medicinally for healing wounds, for sprains and bruises, and for rheumatism; used internally for intestinal problems.

Poisonous principles and symptoms

The plant contains a pigment known as hypericine. This causes a condition known as photosensitisation in which the skin becomes sensitive to sunlight and develops small lesions on its surface. In severe cases the lesions are abraded by the animal which paves the way for infection to set in. Other symptoms of ingestion include loss of appetite, debility, staggering gait and coma. Low level poisoning is probably more common in Britain than is realised. Severe cases have been reported in horses.

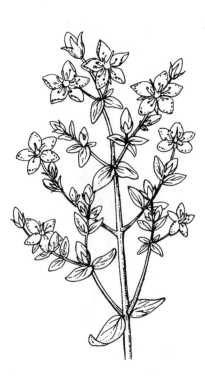

Sorrel (Rumex spp.)

Sheep's sorrel (*Rumex acetosella*) is common throughout Britain on waste and cultivated land and on heaths. Growing up to 30 cm tall, it prefers acid soil and is virtually absent from calcareous land. Common sorrel (*Rumex acetosa* – illustrated) is like sheep's sorrel but larger, sometimes growing up to 100 cm tall. It is more tolerant of chalky soil.

Poisonous principles and symptoms

Whilst other toxic substances such as glycosides are present in both species, ingestion of oxalates is commonly regarded as being their poisonous principle. When animals have become ill after eating the plant, symptoms that were consistent with oxalate poisoning were observed, such as staggering, inabiity to rise, muscular spasm and abnormal breathing. The plants have a taste that is not unattractive to animals and it is often eaten in quantity with no apparent ill effects; the conditions in which poisoning does occur are not clearly defined. There are early reports of horses being poisoned by sorrel but few in modern times.

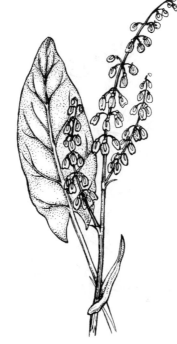

Spurge (Euphorbia spp.)

There are more than 1600 species of spurge, 17 of which occur in Britain. The plant is common on waste and uncultivated land throughout Britain. Spurge takes its name from Euphorbius, physician to King Juba II of Mauritania in A.D. 18. The seeds of *Euphorbia lathyris* (illustrated) were commonly used in medicine of that time as a laxative.

Poisonous principles and symptoms

Many species of spurge contain a milky latex which is thought to be its main toxic principle; there are also resins, glycosides and other toxic substances present in some species. Spurge has caused illness and losses amongst horses in Australia and New Zealand; however, whilst the species of spurge growing in Great Britain are known to be toxic very few cases of poisoning have been reported. Symptoms of poisoning include severe swelling and inflammation of the mouth, salivation and diarrhoea.

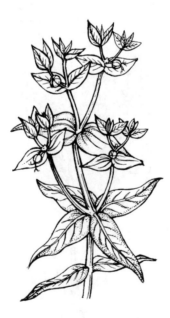

Thorn apple (*Datura stramonium*)

An annual plant preferring waste land, tips, etc., introduced to Europe from its native America. Used in medicine as an antispasmodic and in the homoeopathic treatment of convulsions. An incident at Jamestown in America in the year 1697 gave rise to the common name of the plant, Jimsonweed (Jamestown weed), when soldiers who ate the plant as a vegetable began behaving extremely oddly due to its hallucinogenic properties.

Poisonous principles and symptoms

The thorn apple contains the alkaloids hyoscyamine and hyoscine which are present in all parts of the plant. Symptoms of poisoning may include restlessness, incoordination, dilation of pupils, paralysis and increased respiration rate; death may occur. Poisoning in horses has been reported, although cases are extremely rare, presumably because animals normally find the plant unattractive because of its unpleasant aroma and taste. It is also rarely accessible to horses.

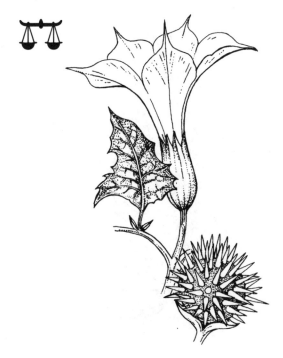

White bryony (Bryonia dioica)

A climbing plant preferring hedges, wet woods, woodland edges, fences and waste ground. Found in west and central Europe; not native in Scotland or western Ireland. White bryony is used in homoeopathy to treat rheumatism. It has a large white root which has been mistaken by people for parsnip or turnip and eaten – with dire consequences. Other common name – British mandrake.

Poisonous principles and symptoms

The poisonous principles of the plant are not clear but they are thought to be associated with a glycoside and an alkaloid. Symptoms of poisoning may include digestive disturbance with acute diarrhoea, profuse urination, profuse sweating, respiratory difficulty, incoordination, convulsions and occasionally cessation of defecation. Affected animals are markedly unwilling to move. Poisoning in horses has been reported.

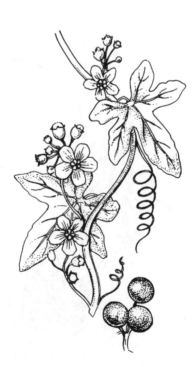

Woody nightshade (*Solanum dulcamara*)

A plant which grows throughout Britain except in some northern areas. Sometimes found on waste ground, but often seen climbing over hedges and woodland trees. A perennial plant which dies back in the winter. It bears oval green berries that turn red when they are ripe. Other common name – Bittersweet.

Poisonous principles and symptoms

All parts of the woody nightshade contain solacine, which is an alkaloidal glycoside. Symptoms of poisoning may include nervous excitement, rapid pulse and respiration, dilated pupils, green diarrhoea, staggering and falling. Poisoning is uncommon and no recent cases have been reported.

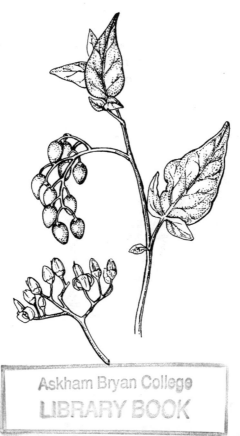

Yew (*Taxus baccata*)

An evergreen tree, native to Britain, growing 20 m in height and preferring chalky soil. It has been cultivated in gardens throughout Britain for centuries. In the past yew was associated with religious ceremonies and very old trees survive in a great many church-yards.

Poisonous principles and symptoms

The yew contains a number of toxic alkaloids which are rapidly absorbed from the digestive tract and affect the action of the heart. The alkaloids are present in all parts of the tree except the fleshy berries (a fact that is contrary to popular belief), and they are not depleted by drying, which makes the clippings particularly haz-ardous to animals. Some confusing information exists concerning the toxic properties of yew, some suggesting that it may be fed as a fodder in some circumstances. However, there is no doubt that it can be fatal especially during the winter months. Symptoms of poisoning include incoordination, coldness, rapid then weak pulse, excitability preceded by collapse. In many cases no symptoms are seen and sudden death occurs within a few hours of ingestion. Many cases of poisoning in horses have been reported.

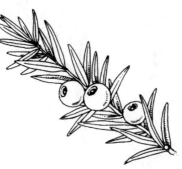

Useful information

Veterinary Poisons Information Unit, National Poisons Information Service (Leeds), Leeds General Infirmary, Great George St, Leeds LS1 3EX. 01132 430715
British Association of Holistic Nutrition and Medicine, Borough Court, Hartley Wintney, Basingstoke, Hants RG27 8JA. 01252 843282.

Index of alternative and Latin names of plants

Other books in the series

A Guide to Equine Nutrition

The case for the return to a more traditional method of keeping and feeding horses based on holistic principles, including a medical assessment and ethical review of materials used in equine feeds and feed additives.

ISBN 0-85131-635-2

A Guide to Herbs for Horses

An informed and impartial explanation of the traditional use of plants and herbs. Essential reading for anyone involved with feeding horses and ponies enabling them to make informed choices about herb-based feeds and supplements.

ISBN 0-85131-646-8

A Guide to Alternative Therapies for Horses

A technically balanced and impartial explanation of the alternative therapies available to the horse owner, which also discusses the underlying principles of the treatments and offers valuable guidance as to who may legally give advice and treatment.

ISBN 0-85131-665-4